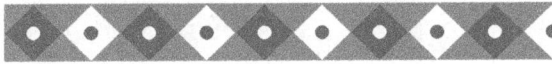

This Book Is Loved...

Trilogy of Cancer: the Jolt, the Journey, the Joy is a small volume which gives a glimpse into some of the thoughts, feelings, creativity, spirit, faith, wisdom, humor, humanness, and wholeness which is personified in Ann Freeman Price. It does so in diversified forms of poetry, prose, chants, and songs (to the tunes of "I've Been Working on the Railroad," "Daisy, Daisy," "Home on the Range," etc.).

If you know Ann, you will see her clearly and hear her profoundly on every page. If you have never had the jolt and joy of being part of a shared journey with her, these images, metaphors, songs, and insights are an introduction to and the gifts of a very wise woman, indeed: psychologically astute, faith-filled and faithful, pain-filled and earthy, honest and real. The words on each page point beyond themselves to the depth and breadth and heights of the complex experience of cancer, surgery, chemotherapy, radiation therapy, re-occurrences, and resurrection experiences of hope, healing, and new life along the way. Perhaps a corollary title could be "A trilogy of living fully, loving deeply, and being all we can be-- regardless of where each of us may be on the journey."

Dr. Charlie McNeil, D.Min., Ed.S., L.M.F.T. and colleague and friend of Ann's.

In its profound simplicity, Ann Freeman Price's poetry captures her cancer experience with grace and precision. Her "Trilogy of Cancer" gives sufferers and their loved ones priceless gifts of candor, comfort and wisdom for their own healing journeys.

Cynthia B. Astle, Editor of United Methodist NeXus. (umnexus.org) and a 10-year cancer survivor.

I have learned over the recent years that no two people ever experience the same cancer. Breast cancer, lymphoma, lung cancer, and, in my case,

This Book Is Loved...

multiple myeloma (and so many more) may all have distinctive medical characteristics yet the groups of people who insurance companies and doctors would like to classify with these similar traits all have their unique cancer and individual experience of their particular disease. This is one of the reasons why I was not quick to search the Internet or read the many books that friends caringly suggested to me in my first months after diagnosis. This was and is my cancer, not someone else's.

Ann Freeman Price, a friend of many decades, gently offered me her own reflections of her experience with cancer, Trilogy of Cancer. It was and continues to be a treasured gift of insight and love. Cancer clearly is a journey and so often we need comfortable and wise traveling companions on the important journeys of our lives. Trilogy of Cancer is one of my companions. It was always close to me for two different and extended stays in the hospital. It was on my bedside table when I returned home after months of chemotherapy.

In sharing aspects of her own journey of cancer, Ann invites the reader, by example not word, to possibly take on aspects of her journey. Reading tiny bits of the Trilogy of Cancer at a time, I found myself taking hold of my life again after handing my body over to a caring, gifted, and learned medical team. Her practices guided much of my early journey in the same way that a traveling companion may make suggestions but the journey is still mine. May your journey be enhanced by Trilogy of Cancer.

The Rev. E. Richard Knox, Ph.D. —-Minister in local parishes and professor of Christian ethics for forty years before his retirement and a person living with cancer.

Ann Freeman Price has a unique voice that sings true on each page. Her personal strength resonates behind her words. This book is a working

This Book Is Loved...

model for those moving through cancer. It embodies spirit, prayer and joy. Price draws the reader into her personal story balancing warmth with candor. Reading these poems, one cannot help but smile in awe at the profound attachment this writer has to life and its complex offerings. Every page is a surprise mixed with wit and intelligence, direction and delight.

Julie Maloney, Director WOMEN READING ALOUD

Ann Freeman Price brings her experience of walking through the challenges of diagnosis, treatment and recovery from cancer to light in this creative and heart warming book. Written in poetic and lyrically flowing style, The Trilogy is a practical and inspiring book that offers insightful perspectives, meaningful insights and innovative suggestions to patients, survivors and caregivers. Using her life-long song writing and spiritual leadership talents, Ann inspires every reader to sing and to celebrate life and live each day to its fullest. The messages are clear and empowering, bringing hope, courage and smiles in ways that can transform times of trial into times of joy.

Lucanne Magill, Assistant Professor, Music Therapy, University of Windsor and formerly Music Therapy Manager, Memorial Sloane Kettering Cancer Center.

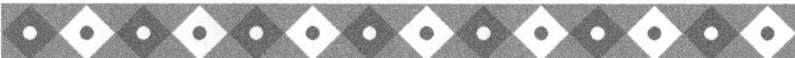

Other books by Ann Freeman Price

Mama & Me: Our Journey Together Her Last Three
Years and Beyond

Wisdom of Children: Questions for God

The Psalms in Shadorma

Do You Love Me? Said the Grandchild to the
Grandma

50 Graces to Sing to Tunes You Know

Woman Songs | Peace Songs Songbook

All books available at: Amazon, Barnes & Noble and
other book sellers.

Music:
Woman Songs | Peace Songs
Available on iTunes and on CD

Signed copies available at:
AnnFreemanPrice.com

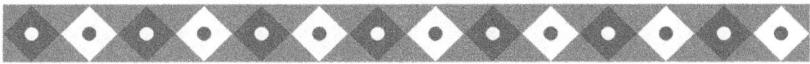

Books In the Works...

Cinderella Smart

Daybook of Personal Faith

To stay up to date on the latest releases visit:

AnnFreemanPrice.com and register!!

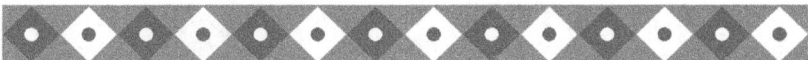

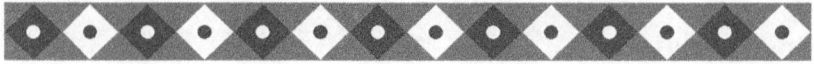

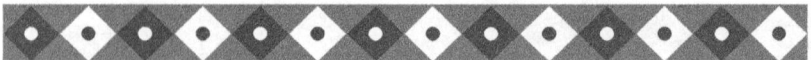

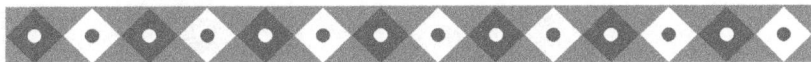

Trilogy of Cancer

The Jolt,
The Journey,
The Joy

Ann Freeman Price

AVIVA
PUBLISHING
New York

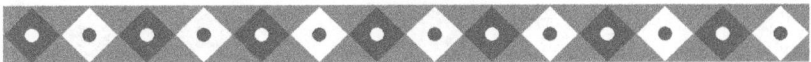

Trilogy of Cancer: The Jolt, The Journey, The Joy
Ann Freeman Price

ISBN #: 978-1-943164-93-6

Published By:
Aviva Publishing
Lake Placid, NY
518-523-1320

Copyright filed with the Library of Congress:
December 20, 2007
September 7, 2018

Design and Layout: Donna L. Price,
Compass Rose Consulting, LLC.
www.compassroseconsulting.com

Artwork:
Emily Bittner, Enchanted-Image
www.Enchanted-Image.com

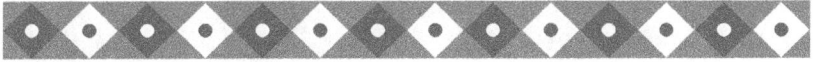

Dedicated to:
  -those who have died of cancer
  -those who survive it
  -those who are caregivers

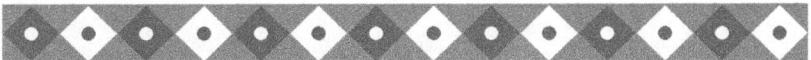

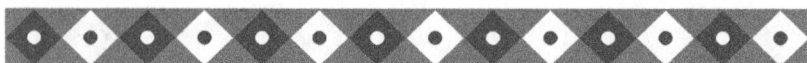

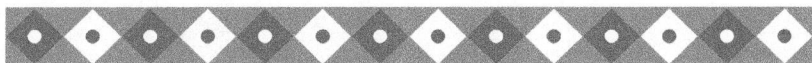

Table of Contents

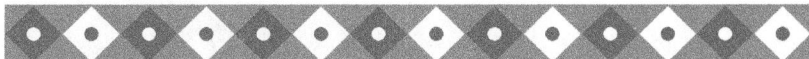

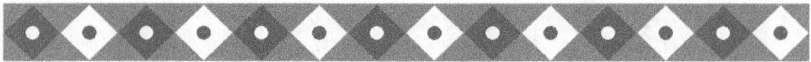

Table of Contents

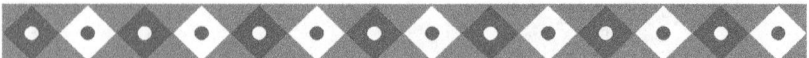

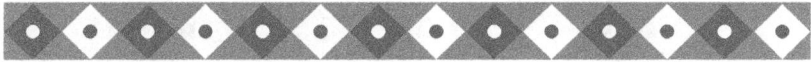

Table of Contents

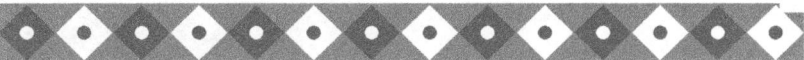

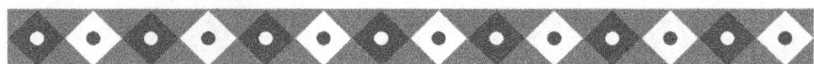

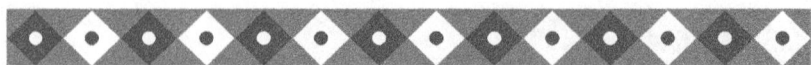

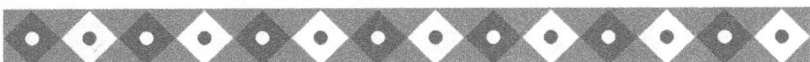

Preface

I am a breast cancer survivor, diagnosed in December 2003. I had surgery, one-time radiation, and three months of chemotherapy---all between January and July of 2004.

The poems, songs, and how-to's in this book tell part of the story of the road I walked.

Soon after surgery, my friend Jeff called to see how I was doing, and as we talked he said, "I can hardly wait to hear the song, because I can't think of a single word that rhymes with 'lumpectomy'."

And the project began.

I used folk tunes for the songs so that others could easily sing them and feel the humor and the truths in their own voices.

In addition to the medical model, I used every alternative I could find that seemed to fit me and work for me---visualization, massage, music, drumming.

I believe each person has to find his or her own road through cancer---and out to the other side of cancer. For me it started with---

The Jolt---Even though each time you have a mammography and you know cancer could be a possibility, I never thought it would be true for me. And then came---

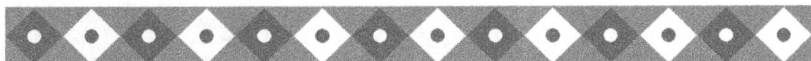

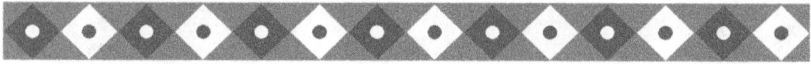

The Journey---It seemed like I moved from one decision to another with relatively little time to research. I called people I knew. They referred me to people I didn't know. I talked and listened. I decided what to do, and did it---with enormous support. And now comes---

The Joy---Actually the joy was tucked into every part but it certainly vibrates in a very strong way now.

The three really interweave. There are no absolutely clear division lines. Sometimes even the jolt pops up now, as I find myself telling someone that I had breast cancer and I hear a small voice inside me saying "Really? Did you?" And the jolt is there again.

Actually I got the jolt two more times because this is a revision of the first book. Two more lumps in the same breast—and the story is here—read it all and figure out what you can fit into your experience.

If this trilogy resonates with you; if some song helps you stand tall and breathe deep; if a poem encourages you to smile; if a how-to inspires you to try a new way---then the trilogy is working.

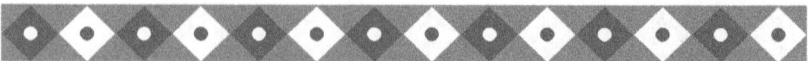

And on top of all that, a portion of the proceeds of this book goes to a cancer program. I wrote a simple song for the Sussex County Relay for Life and one of the verses said,

> Sometimes I forget that it's partly up to me
> To keep walkin', to keep talkin' for a cure,
> Yes, sometimes I forget that it's partly up to me
> To keep the pressure on for a cure.

Some of us have joined a club which we didn't want to join and when the cure is found, eventually the Cancer Club won't need to exist anymore.

Ann Freeman Price

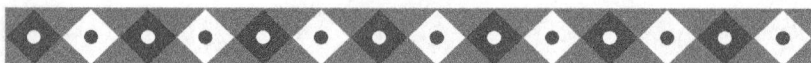

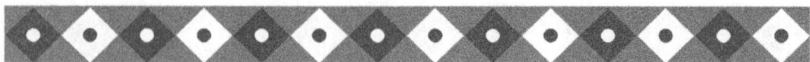

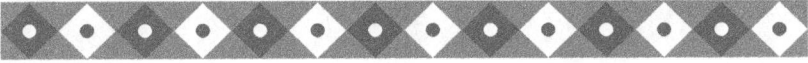

The Jolt

Diagnosis
&
Surgery

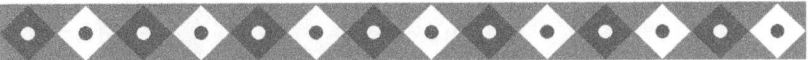

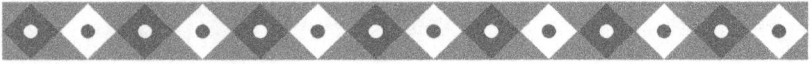

Routine

some things are
routine
changing your sheets
cleaning the house
getting a tune-up
for the car
getting the mammography
each year

they say they need
more pictures...
still routine

they say they need
an ultrasound...
still routine

they say they need
a needle biopsy...

stop
where are
we going

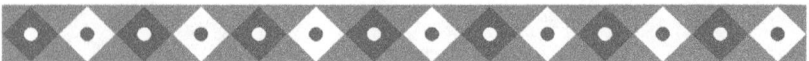

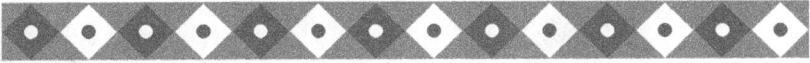

they say to call
after three on Monday

they say
it's breast cancer

I want to
go back
to routine

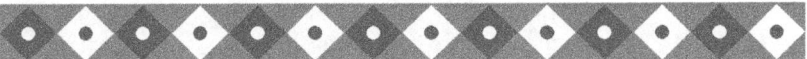

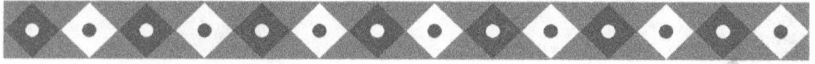

Tell Them What to Say

I told them
what to say
in surgery
> nurse
>
> surgeon
>
> anesthesia person

at beginning
please say
"you will heal
very well"

in middle
say "you're
doing great"

toward end
say "you'll
wake up and
things will
go as they
should"

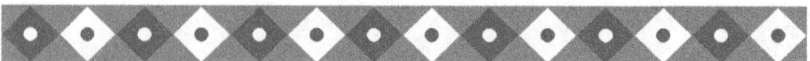

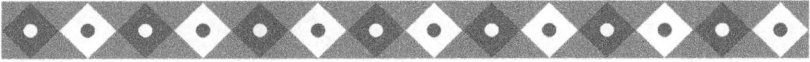

they said them
I healed well
I did great

things went
as they should

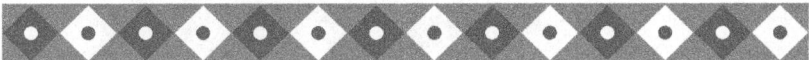

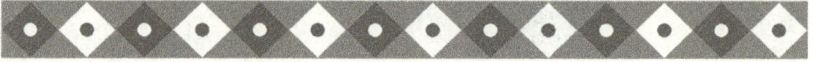

This Drain-O!

I'll be glad, yes I'll be glad
      when I don't have this drain-O!
It is nothing, it is nothing
      but a big old pain-O!
When we empty it each day
      There is not a doubt-O
We'll be glad when this old drain
      Is ready to come out-O!

(Sing to the tune: Yankee Doodle)

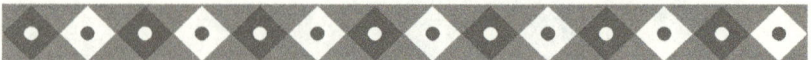

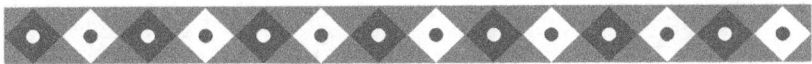

This Drain-O!

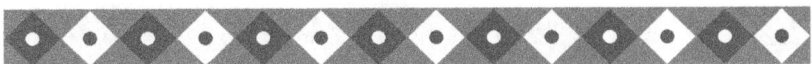

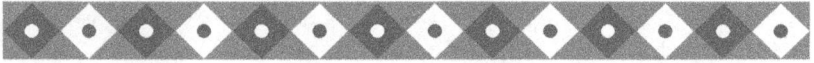

Oh, Lump-ec-to-my!

O sing me a song
'Bout a day that went wrong
When they did the lumpectomy.
Well the nodes were bad too
So they took out a few
And two scars for Ann you can see.
　　　Oh, lumpectomy,
　　　It's a pain and that I'll agree.
　　　So let's move on right now,
　　　I'll be showin' you how
　　　We're gonna be findin' a key.

(Sing to the tune: Home on the Range)

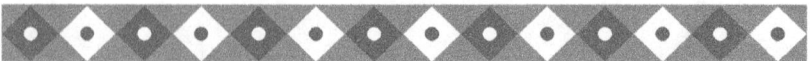

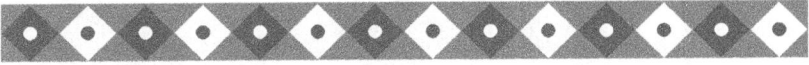

Oh Lumpectomy

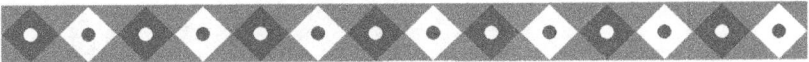

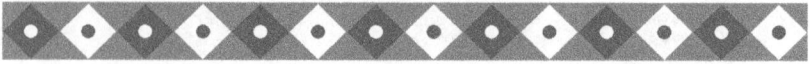

How to---Prepare for Surgery

There is a book titled "Prepare for Surgery---Heal Faster" by Peggy Huddleston. I got the book just a couple of days before my surgery and after skimming it, called their office and received a phone number where I could make arrangements for some training in their system over the phone.

I did that and talked on the phone for a little over two hours. The only cost to me was the phone call.

In that time we went over the things I would ask the people in the operating room to say to me when I was unconscious.

They asked me to decide on a comfort image. This would be an image that I would ask friends and family to visualize and that I would imagine for myself. I chose to be wrapped and held in a yellow blanket of love.

In the phone conversation, the trainer asked me to tell her what I would be doing in six months, one year, five years. I thought and then told her and wrote them down---all ways of planting those pictures in my brain.

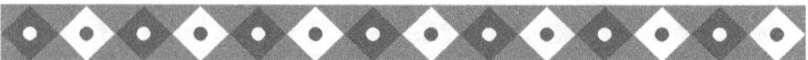

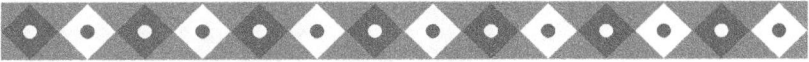

I found it helpful---both in terms of getting through the surgery in a very positive way, and in terms of giving family and friends a way to support me and be helpful.

There is a website: www.healfaster.com
There is a phone number: 781-864-2668

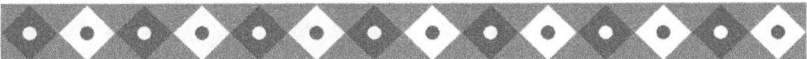

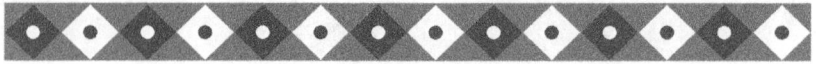

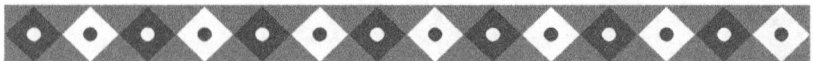

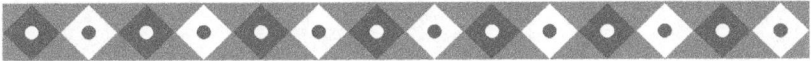

The Journey

Radiation

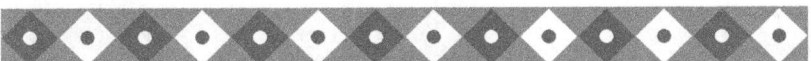

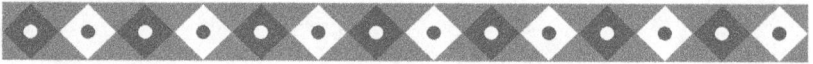

Pioneer

they said
you'll be a
pioneer

this one-time
radiation

new thing
part of a
study

I thought of
wagons crossing
prairies
wild animals
attacking

I said
I'm not a
pioneer

then I
researched

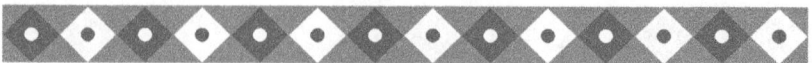

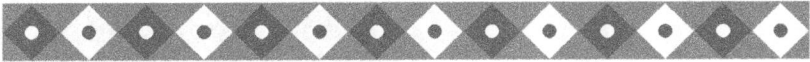

radiation the
usual way

five days a week
for six weeks

I closed
my eyes
and saw
some wagons
arriving safely
sturdy women
and men
building homes
raising children

I said
OK

where do I
sign to be
a pioneer

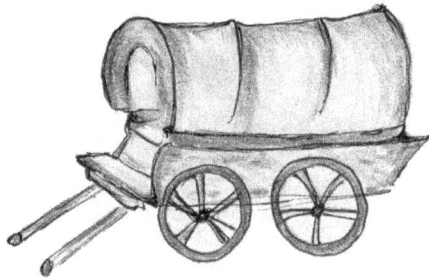

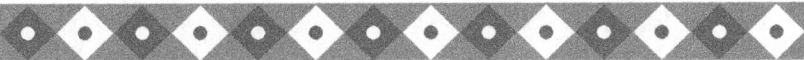

Yellow Blanket and Daffodils

what do you
want to be
wrapped in
she asked

I thought
and then
spoke clearly
to trainer

yellow
I want to be
wrapped in a
soft yellow
blanket

I spread the word
among friends
family
pastor

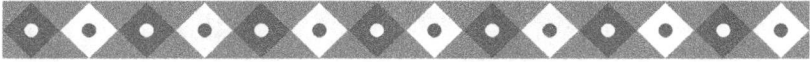

during surgery
think of me
see me held
in yellow blanket

I dreamed of
softness, I saw
the yellow and
felt the love
and warmth

we traveled
two hours
to hospital
arriving at much
too early hour
of six a.m.

once checked in
they waved us
toward waiting room
we'll call you
when it's time

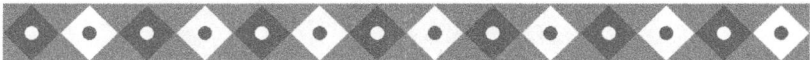

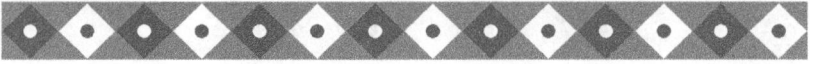

we paused at edge of
large room stuffed
with many sofas
perched between
end tables

each table held
a vase of yellow
jonquils in January

it
works

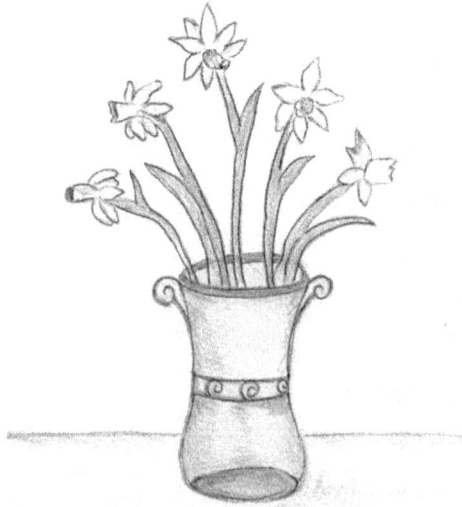

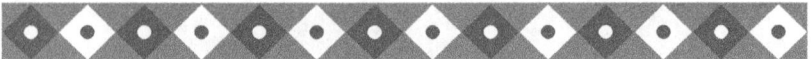

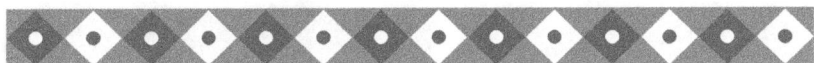

The Journey

Healing Ways

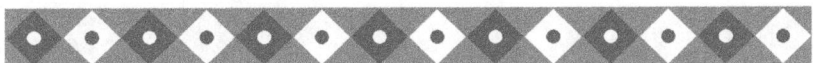

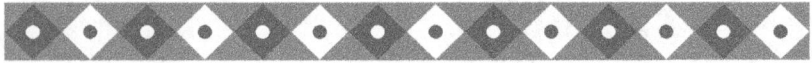

Healing Circle

we gathered
in a circle
just before
the chemo start

friends and family
brought themselves
complete with concern
to sit in support

some held
within themselves
the faith
of decades

some sat
with hope
and doubt
stirred together
in a batter
that resists
the mixing

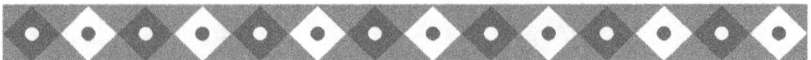

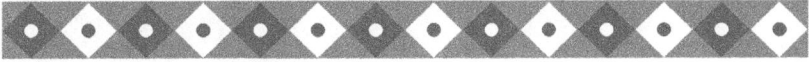

we sang
and dreamed
together of
wholeness

they wrote
their prayers
on colored
circles

one side
their prayer
for me

other side
someone
within their
life who needed
my prayers
as I sat for
chemo in
weeks to come

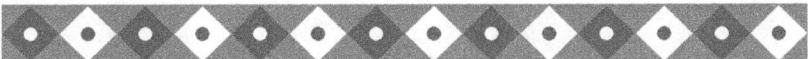

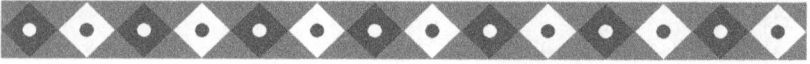

we prayed
and loved
within this
circle of healing

which ended
at a time

and yet
goes on
in time

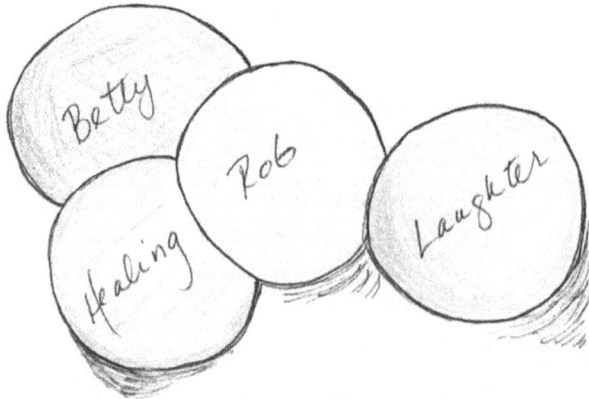

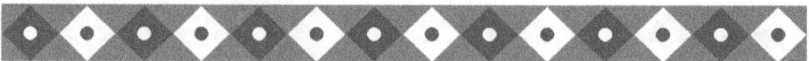

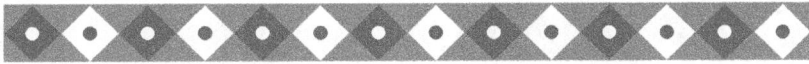

35 Squares

afghan squares
knit with needles
yarn and love

varied colors weave
through multi-patterns
each one different

squares made by
women creating
with skill and prayer

I sit in cubical for
chemo and afghan
lies on lap

chemicals drip
through needles, prayer love
flows through afghan

who knows which
pierced the cancer
probably love

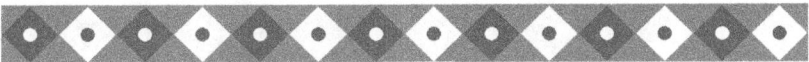

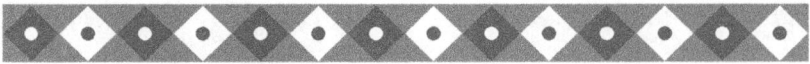

Circling 'Round

Circling round are prayers and lovingness,
Prayers and lovingness,
Circling round is faith unending, yes!
Faith unending, yes!
Circling, healing, loving.

Circling round is music vibrating,
Music vibrating,
Circling round is touch with energy,
Touch with energy,
Circling, healing, loving.

Circling round are friends and family,
Friends and family,
Circling round are hands a-holding me,
Hands a-holding me,
Circling, healing, loving.

(Sing to the tune: O How Lovely Is the Evening)

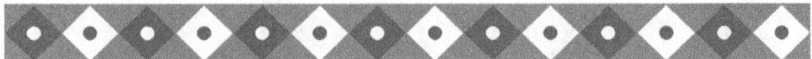

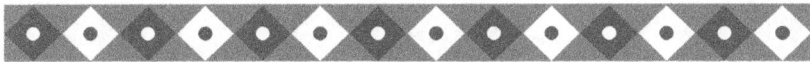

Circling 'Round

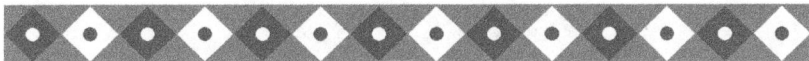

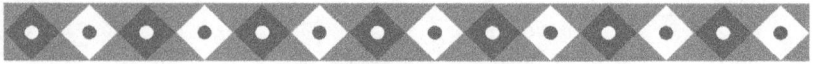

Chemo Notebook

a poem
joke
prayer
story
wish

request went
out "send me
something that
I can sit with"

they sent them
favorite quotes
words to songs
pictures of
peace and healing
for chemo notebook

mail increased
and each went
into the three-ring
binder
unread

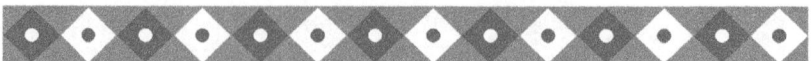

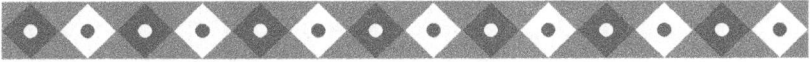

save it for later
and savor it then

hours of chemo
crawled some days
but time still went
faster with the
notebook

with each reading
came a friend
to sit with me
a while
caring
hoping
praying

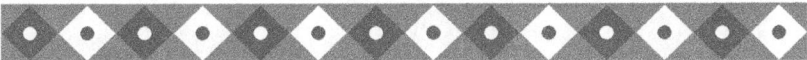

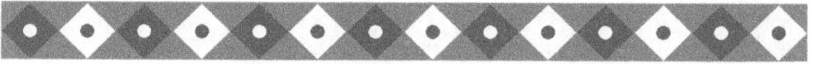

How to—-Have a Healing Circle

There's certainly no right or wrong way to have a healing circle.

I held the circle on the day before I started chemo. I invited family members, close friends, and anyone from my church who wanted to come.

Here are some of the ingredients that we used:

Candle lighting---Candles are important to me, so we lit them.

Music---my daughter taught the beginning song and I taught the ending one. I used a Native American chant: "O Great Spirit---earth, sun, sky and sea---you are inside---and all around me."

My speaking---I thanked them each for coming and told them that my mind's picture for this chemo trip was going to be of water---cleansing, clear, wonderful water, and that I would think of that as I had the chemo.

Visualization---The pastor led a visualization exercise, using my image of water, moving, cascading, cleaning.

Others speaking---There was a chance for each person in the circle who wanted to speak about their hopes for me.

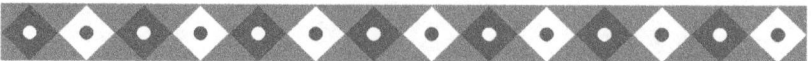

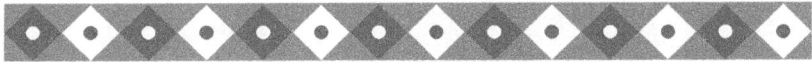

Writing on the circles---We provided a 3-inch circle for each person and on one side they wrote their prayer for me. On the other side they wrote about someone they knew that they would like me to pray for. I took these circles with me each time to chemo---read their prayers for me, and prayed for the people they asked me to pray for.

It was probably 45 minutes and a wonderful time for me of support, of surrounding, of presence.

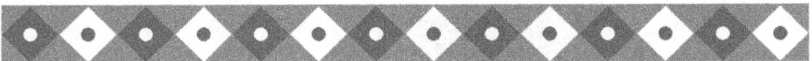

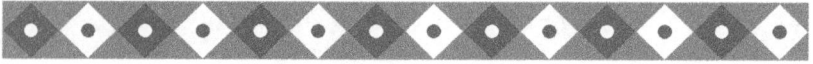

How to—-Have a Chemo Notebook

I knew that chemo would take time.

I wanted to take friends with me---even those far away.

So I sent out an email and wrote, "Send me something for my chemo notebook I'm making. Send me your favorite poem or story or picture or prayer. I won't look at it ahead of time. But during chemo I'll read what you send. It will pass the time and better still it will connect me with you."

The contributions came in the mail. They went into the notebook---and I did not read them. And when I went to chemo, it worked just as I hoped it would.

Some things they had sent were funny---some were nostalgic memories---some were serious and thoughtful.

I portioned them out so that they would last the entire three months.

And they connected me with friends---with family.

And they took me beyond myself.

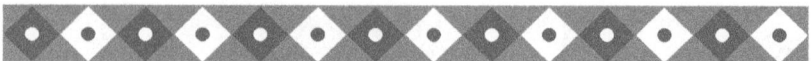

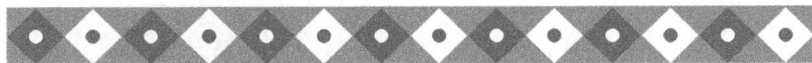

The Journey

Chemotherapy

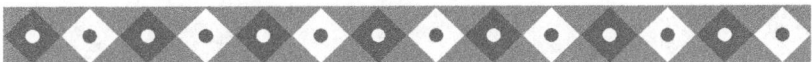

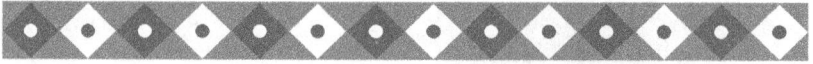

Oh Dear!

Oh dear, Doctor says it's cancer,
Dear, dear, Doctor says it's cancer,
Oh dear, Doctor says it's cancer,
Now we'll come up with a plan.

> So first we'll have surgery, then radiation,
> And then chemotherapy, what a sensation,
> We'll take old tamoxifen, five years the ration,
> And then I'll write more songs like this.

So it's oh dear, cancer is not winning
No, dear, cancer is not winning,
My dear, cancer is not winning,
'Cause I came up with a plan.

> I'll go on the breast cancer walks far as I can go,
> Wear my pink bracelet so other survivors know,
> Offer support to a friend in the club who's low,
> Then I'll write more songs like this.

Now it's, Hey you, let me tell you the news,
Yes, you, let me tell you the news,
You, You---let me tell you the news:
You must come up with a plan.

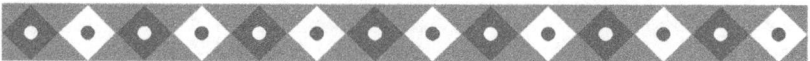

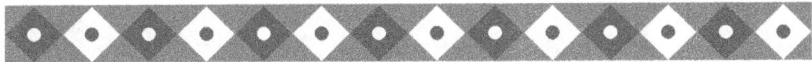

You need once a year to go get a mammography,

Don't put it off, just go get a mammography,

Get in your car and go get a mammography,

Then I'll write more songs like this!

(Sing to the tune: Oh Dear, What Can the Matter Be?)

Oh Dear

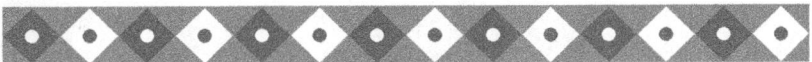

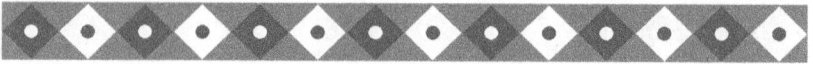

Chemotherapy: Part 1

I am sleeping,

I am sleeping,

'Cause I hurt,

'Cause I ache,

Chemo makes me frown,

Chemo wears me down,

Sleep on through,

Sleep on through.

(Sing to the tune: Are You Sleeping, Brother John?)

(Sing slowly)

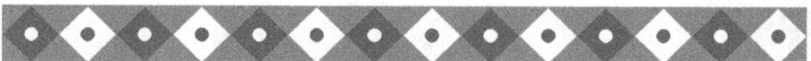

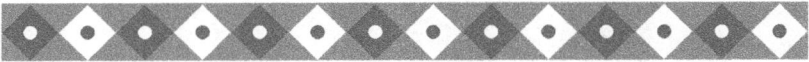

The Hair

Oh where, oh where has my pretty hair gone?
Oh where, oh where could it be?
When it first fell out, I just shaved it off bald
And now I wear hats you see.

(Sing to the tune: Oh Where, Oh Where Has My Little
Dog Gone?)

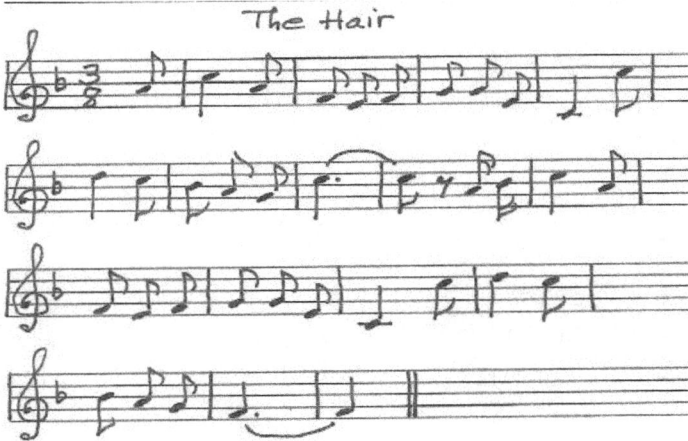

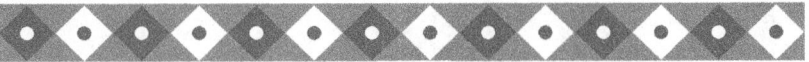

The Hair

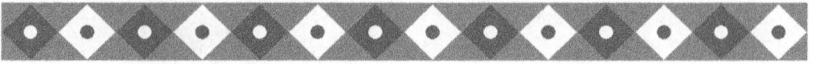

Ga?

she stood at the
foot of the bed
three years old with
bangs partly covering
the concern mapped
on her forehead

chemo was
taking its toll
scuttling any effort
on my part to get up
and greet or
meet the day

my eyes
drifted open
and I saw her

her hand patted
the bed cover
and she asked
"Ga?" (short for
Grandma?) "Are
you still not
feeling well?"

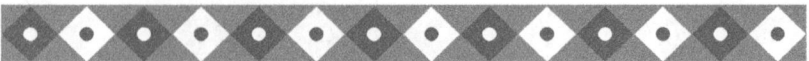

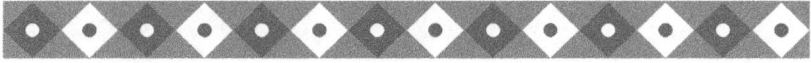

Not Coney Island

I never did like
roller coaster rides
and never planned
to buy a ticket
for the chemo one

but I'm on it
and as I leave
today's treatment
I ride the
straight away

the steroids
keep it steady
as clock ticks
through first day
first night and
then without ever
climbing up
the descent begins

no thrill
in this ride

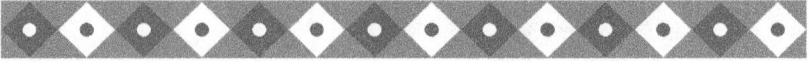

I start my plunge with
muscle collapse
no appetite
aches
tired
all the way down

continuing days
ask how far down
can this ride go

then somewhere
it turns

baked potatoes
taste good
muscles let go
of their ache
small spurts of energy
begin to build

the roller coaster
is climbing up

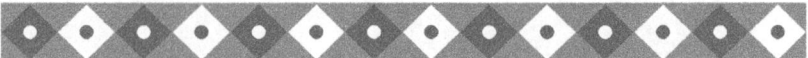

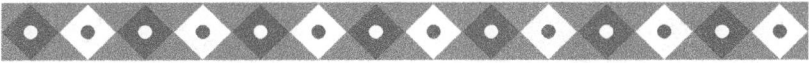

skies brighten
the clack of wheels
clatter in time with
my heart hopes

two weeks have
passed and here
almost at the
top I sit in
coaster car
poised...

for next
chemo day

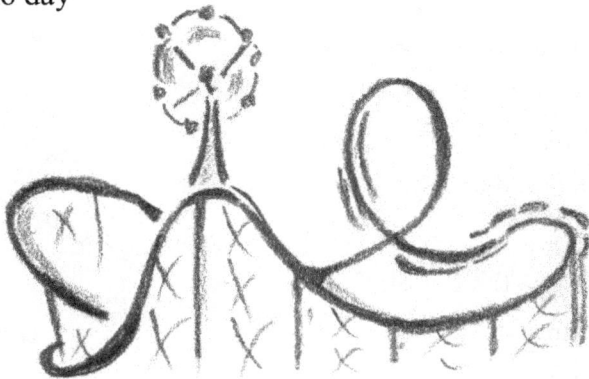

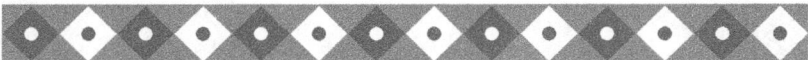

Cleaning Out

years ago my
friend asked her
Cherokee mother
about her constant
wellness

and when I
faced chemo
same friend called
to tell me of her
mother's scrubbly
bubbles remedy

lie down and open
the bottoms of your feet
let in the scrubbly
bubbles and close your
feet tight again

move the bubbles
through your body
up legs around knees
let them bubble wherever

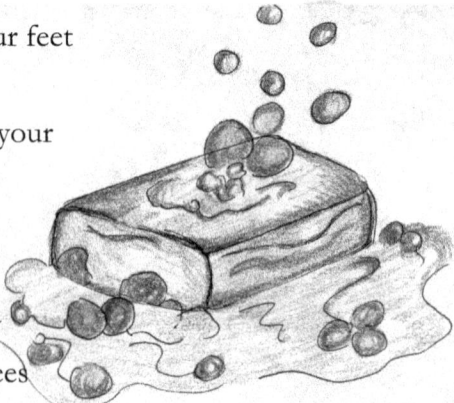

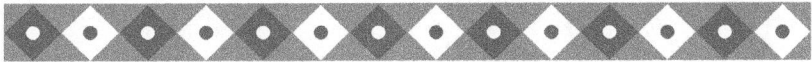

you feel pain
and need

up your body
into your hips
scrubble throughout
your bloodstream

swish around your
breast let bubbles
heal and cleanse
into your arms
out to the tips
scrubbling commence
where nodes were
taken out

bubble into your neck
wash away tense muscles
bubble through
chemo drugs

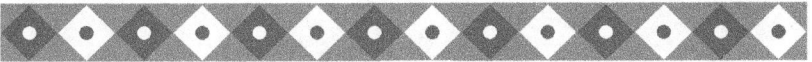

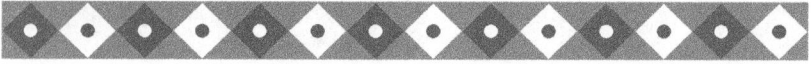

bubble into your head
clean your brain
of fear and question

as scrubbly bubbles
finish open the top
of your head and
let them out
carrying with them
the pain and poison
the ache of tension
the fear and worry

I listened
and I did it
over and over

they did no harm
those scrubbly bubbles

passed down through
generations and cultures
they may have
done good

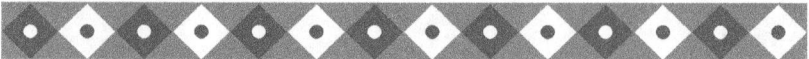

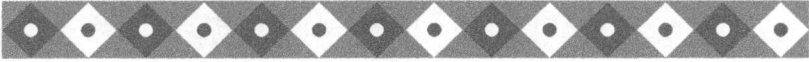

I Decide

I marched in
halfway through
three months of
treatments and
said with authority
"You said Taxol
would be easier.
It isn't."

they listened

"Today" my voice
was clear "Today
I want copies of
everything: blood
pressure, temperature,
blood work numbers
Everything"

they gave them
to me

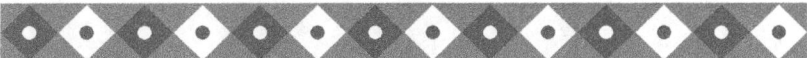

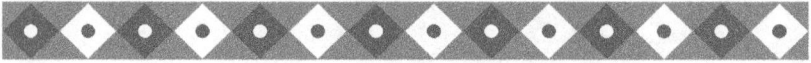

"Today is different"
I told calm doctor
as if he didn't know
"You tell me if it's
a 'go' for today's
treatment

but then you need
to sell me again
on why I'm
doing this

give me statistics
name my options
say your best judgment

and then
then I'll decide
if it's a 'go'"

he did that

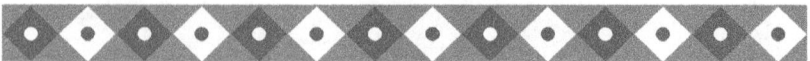

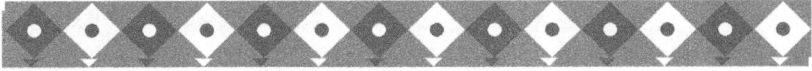

I decided to
keep going
but on that day
I claimed strength
and power and
control

I never let go
of them again

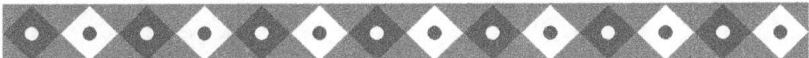

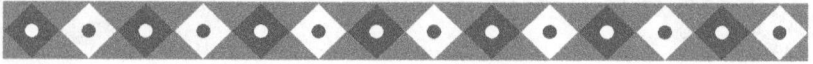

In Charge

I will not permit
Breast cancer to win,
I will live every day
Relishing each new way
I can put a spin----

On the time I have,
Every golden hour,
Whether there's thunder
Or rainstorms or sun
I will have the power----

To give out a smile
To a friend or foe,
I will stay positive
Most of the life I live
Everywhere I go!!!

(Sing to the tune: Row, Row, Row Your Boat)

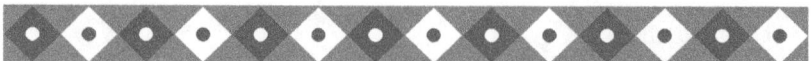

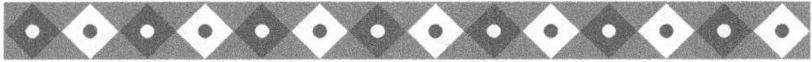

In Charge

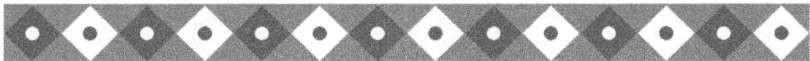

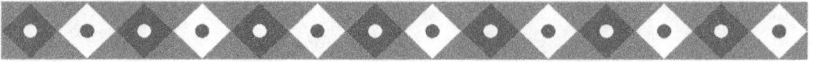

Chemotherapy: Part 2

We'll sit down and get the chemotherapy
We'll sit down and get the chemotherapy
Swallow pills and watch the drip,
Chemotherapy's a trip,
We'll sit down and get the chemotherapy.
> Steroids keep the vomiting suppressed for now,
> Steroids keep the vomiting suppressed for now,
> But when those old steroids wear off,
> You will ache and pain and swear off,
> Steroids keep the vomiting suppressed for now,

Then you start to feel yourself again at last,
Then you start to feel yourself again at last,
But it's not a four-leaf clover,
'Cause it's time to start all over,
Even though you feel yourself again at last.
> Where's the word, oh where's the word, it's
> > "chemo brain!"
> Where's the word, oh where's the word, it's
> > "chemo brain!"
> They all say "Slow down, don't hurry,"
> They all say "Just don't you worry,"
> Where's the word, oh where's the word, it's
> > "chemo brain!"

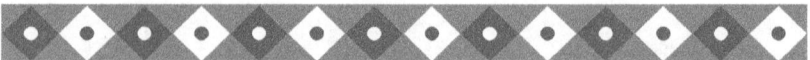

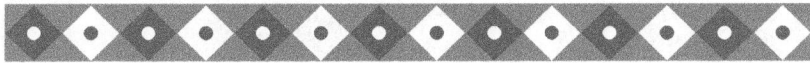

Chemo's done, Oh Chemo's done, Do you believe?

Chemo's done, Oh Chemo's done, Do you believe?

Let's all stand and shout hooray!

Never thought we'd see this day!

Chemo's done, Oh chemo's done, Yes I believe!!!

(Sing to the tune: She'll Be Comin' Around the Mountain)

Chemotherapy: Part 2

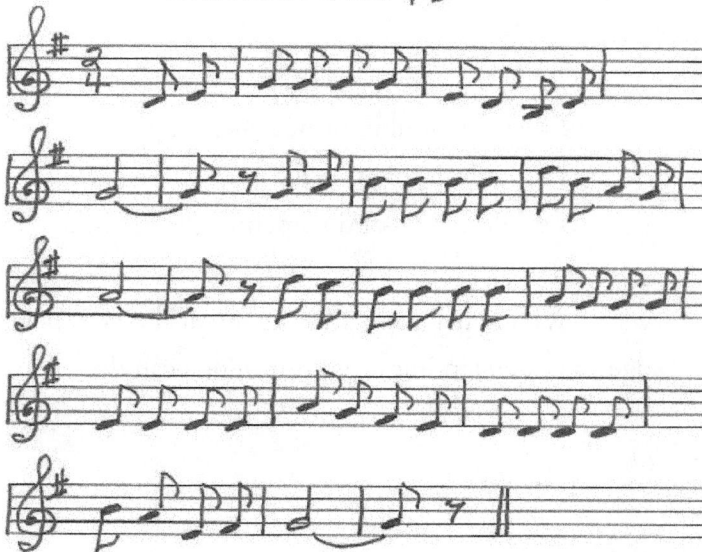

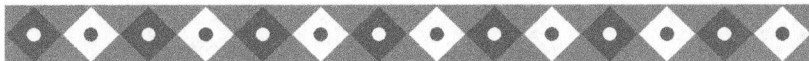

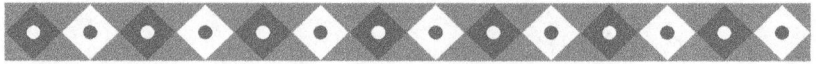

How to—-Scrubbly Bubbles

In some ways the poem says it all. I had started chemo when my friend called and told me of how her mother seemed to never be sick. When she asked her about it, her mother (Cherokee Indian) told her about scrubbly bubbles.

Basically it's visualization. It's imagining opening the bottom of your feet and letting the bubbles in. It's visualizing those bubbles moving throughout your body in a systematic way. It's letting them bubble and cleanse and move on. And then it's seeing in your mind's eye opening the top of your head and letting the bubbles out again.

> I knew it would not hurt anything.
> I thought it might help.
> I think it did---and sometimes I still do it.

What I believe is that we are at the very beginning edge of understanding what our minds can do.

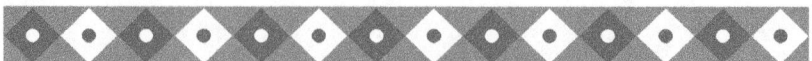

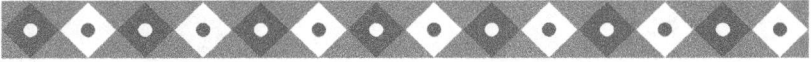

Throughout these cancer treatments, I challenged myself and others to do things. I asked the surgeon to talk to me and say specific things during surgery. I thought of myself wrapped in a yellow blanket and asked other people to do the same. I imagined the bubbles.

Throughout, I put myself on that edge and said, "Let's try out this mind and body thing. It can't hurt. I think it can help."

I believe it did.

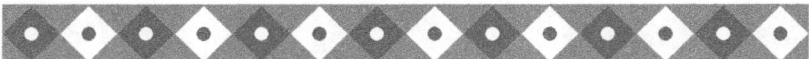

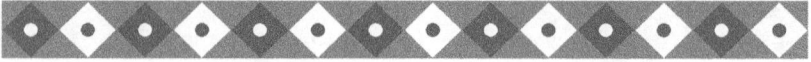

How to—-Stay in Charge

I believe that staying in charge is a decision-based action.

It's deciding that you are the authority on your body and on your self.

And then it's communicating that.

I was looking forward to Taxol because they said it would be an easier drug to tolerate. And I was angry when it wasn't. For me, it was worse.

So I went in---spurred by my anger.

But I came out---feeling free. I felt like I did in fact know best. I knew my body. I knew what was best for me.

And even though I decided to continue the course of chemo treatment, I did it in a new way.

I felt the newness, and I believe that the doctors and nurses felt it too.

And that reality---of me being in charge of what was going to happen next---made a difference in the rest of the treatment---and makes a difference in the rest of my life!

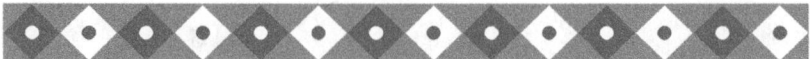

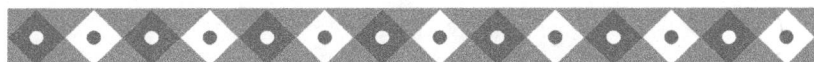

The Joy

After Chemo

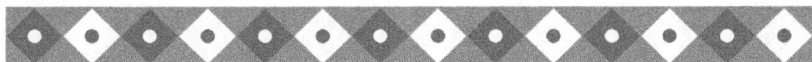

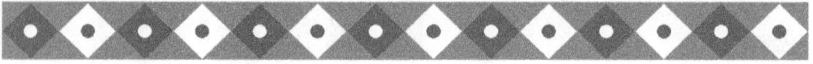

Prayers Present

the prayers
never leave
never arrive
just are

prayers present
in the surrounding
in the loving

prayers pulsing
in fingers of massage
in vibration of drum

prayers active
in words of caring
in warmth of afghan

no asking prayers
with answers
of yes or no

but holding prayers
where God says so clearly
"I will never
let you go"

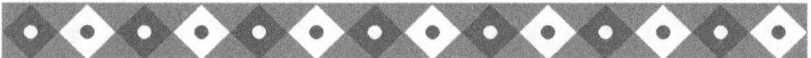

The Bracelet

it was October
Breast Cancer Month

he was seventeen
his aunt died of it
his grandmother
survives it

"where's a pink
bracelet?" he asked

"I have extras"
his mother told him

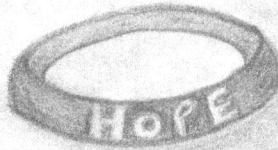

"I need one"
"Why?"
"to wear---it's
October!"

"you'll wear it
to school? pink?"

"it's October
I'll wear it"

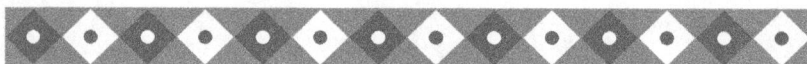

Cancer

Cancer, Cancer

Do not come back to me,

I'm quite happy

Living so cancer free,

I will not spend time in worry,

I can't afford that flurry,

But I do know

That if it shows

I will deal with it

And just be !!

(Sing to the tune: Daisy, Daisy)

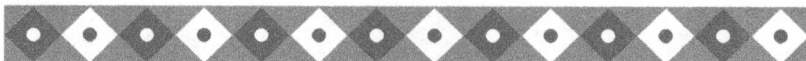

60

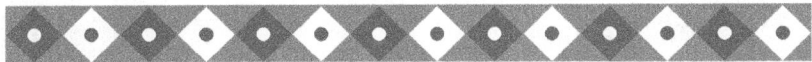

The Pink Walk

once a year
we walk
thousands of us

some walk
to honor those
who didn't
make it

some walk
to celebrate
the ones who did

some walk
and wear survivor
shirts and show
thumbs up
in passing

raise more money
raise awareness
remind each other
to mammo each year

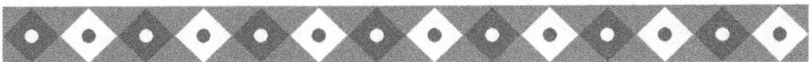

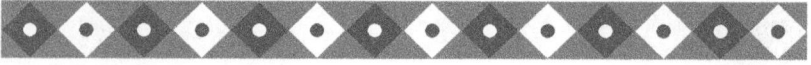

and as we walk
we wonder when
breast cancer
will be disease
of past

for now
we walk

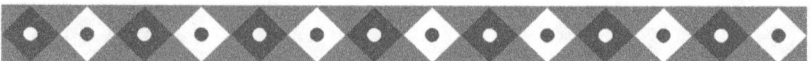

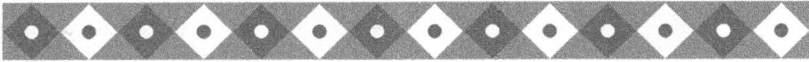

Feel the Drum

Feel the drum, Feel the drum,

Deep inside, Deep inside,

Now as you are beating the drums don't you see

Vibrations are traveling from drum back to me

And cells that were scattered are suddenly free to

Feel the drum.

(Sing to the tune: Three Blind Mice)

Feel the Drum

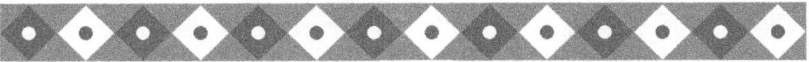

63

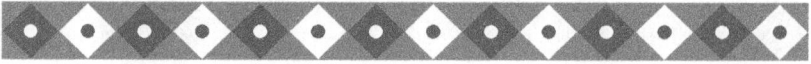

Healing Drum

simple hand drum
steady beat
five minutes
a day

five minutes
to feel my hand
touch skin of drum
synchronize with
heart and blood

five minutes for
cancer cells
to scatter from
the pounding
and the pulsing
of the ancient sound

five minutes
to feel vibration
connecting cell to cell
organizing life stream

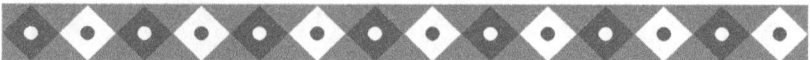

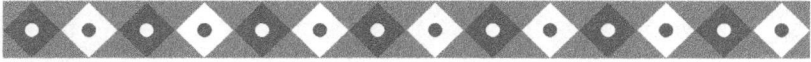

five minutes
for beat and breath
to gather energy
for the day

the day which
starts with
drumming

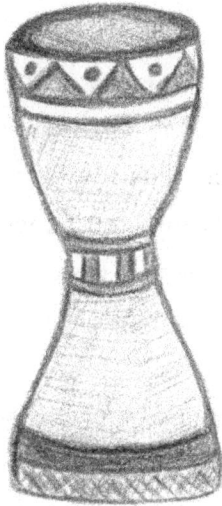

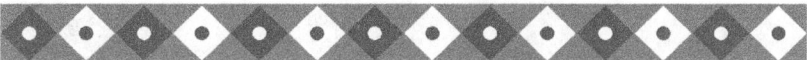

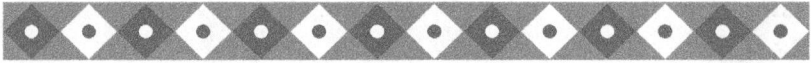

How to— Play the Drum

I am no master drummer.

I can only give a "how to" on this one, based on my experience.

I am a music therapist and in my training at New York University, I was in a music therapy group at the same time that my mother died. I remember going to group several days after her death and at some point sitting myself behind the big drum. As I drummed, I felt it pulling some of the scattered pieces of my self back together. I experienced the vibration working within my body, permeating the feelings, piercing the cells, pounding into my breath.

I didn't actually start using the drum in the midst of cancer. I started it two years after chemo. I play five minutes a day and I plan to play at least that much every day for the rest of my life. If I were to have cancer again, I would just keep playing the drum.

I beat a rhythm, I breathe deeply, I feel my hands against the skin of the drum. I speak to it---sometimes chant, sometimes just sing tones---and the drum speaks back.

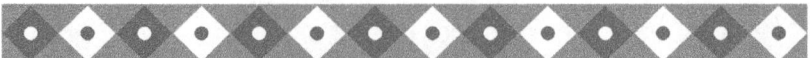

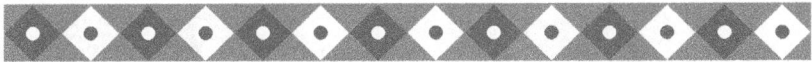

The Joy

Living

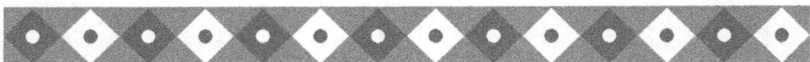

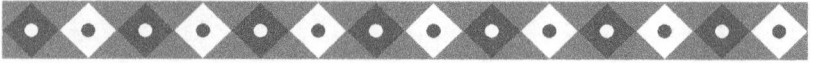

The Gifts of Winter

I barely remember
those January days
when into the cold
and brand new year I carried
the news that was itself
just barely two weeks old
the news of cancer---"biopsy
of left breast is positive"

"Damn" I whispered
into the frigid wind
"Damn" I shouted
onto slippery streets
"How dare the flakes
of snow drift down
as if there is no
one thing changed"

we made the plans
that had to be made
---the surgery---
---new one-time radiation---

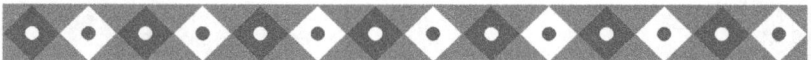

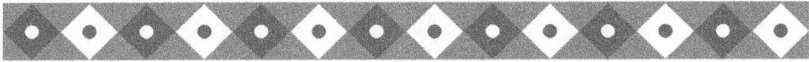

we skidded to hospital
and home again

it was my least
favorite season
even if you did not
factor in cancer

but that winter
now three years past
that winter
gave its gifts

of healing
in the middle of chill

of surrounding love
in the middle of ice

of promise of life
in the edges of spring

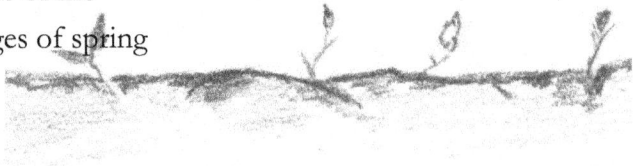

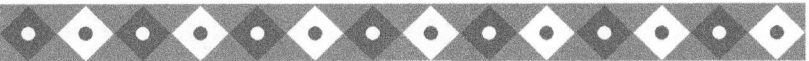

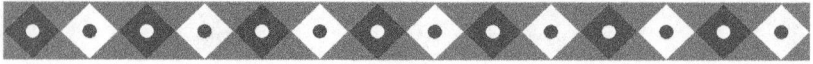

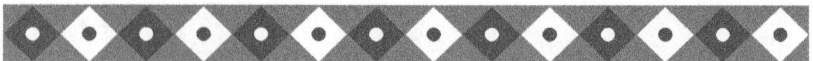

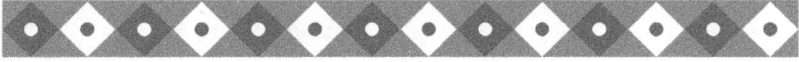

Oops
Take Two-
And Three

More Surgery

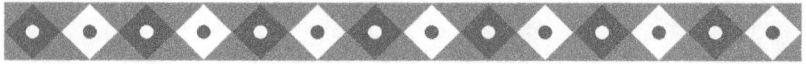

Dump Lumps

Cancer-free for ten years,
A decade of remission
And then returns a tiny lump
Ready for excision.

Two years more — another lump,
This time drastic measure
Remove one breast and radiate
The place of former treasure.

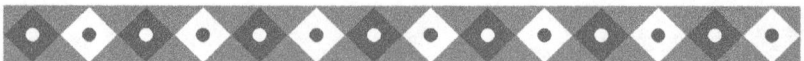

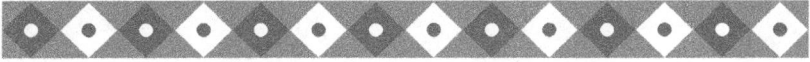

Three Times

I had breast cancer once,
I had breast cancer twice,
But when they found it the third time
They said, "This isn't nice."

So now I have one breast,
Yes, now I have one breast,
And that will do to see me through,
Yes, now I have one breast.

(Sing to the tune: The Farmer in the Dell)

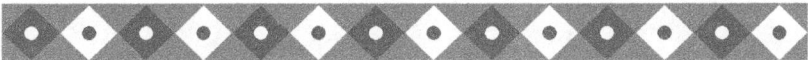

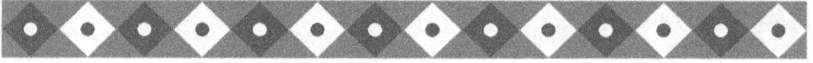

Yo!

Yo! Check out the mirror!
Something significant is missing here.

Yo! Now I see beneath bruises and stitches
I have clearly lost one of my riches.

Yo! What does it mean? How shall I cope
The same way as always, you silly old dope.

Yo! One breast or two, two breasts or one
You're still the same person and the deed it is done.

Yo! Check out the mirror!

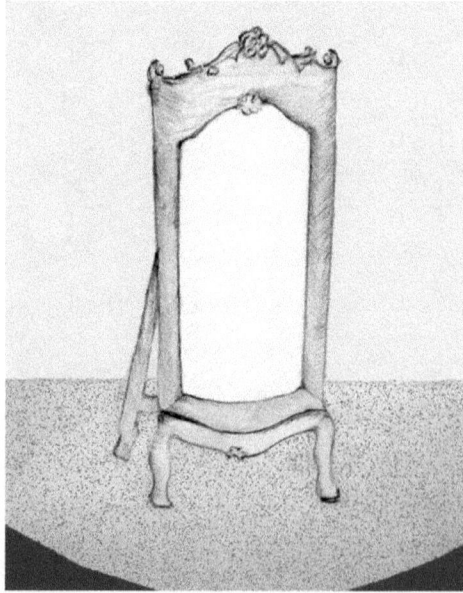

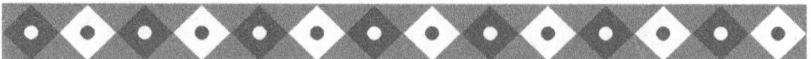

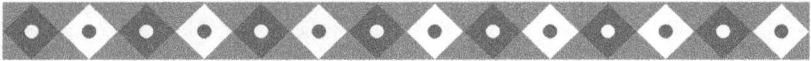

Radiation

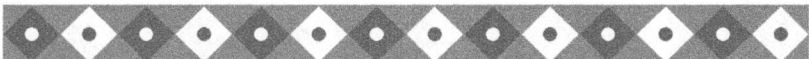

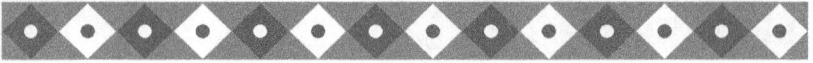

Rays of Healing

Rays of radiation into
Rays of healing,
Let it be
on this day,
let it be.

Rays of radiation into
Rays of healing,
Let it be
on this day,
let it be.

As I lie down
covered in prayer,
help me know that
God is there turning
Rays of radiation into
Rays of healing,
Let it be
on this day,
let it be.

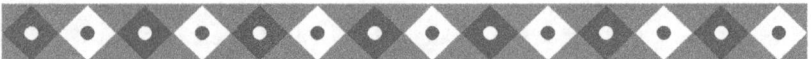

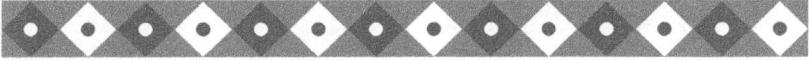

Don't Delay

Well I laid right down to get the rays
Singin' gonna beat the cancer today.
Well I laid right down to get the rays
Singin' gonna beat the cancer today.

Get it done! Get it done!
Get it done and don't delay,
Every one I do will see me through,
Singin' gonna beat the cancer today.

(Sing to the tune: Polly Wolly Doodle)

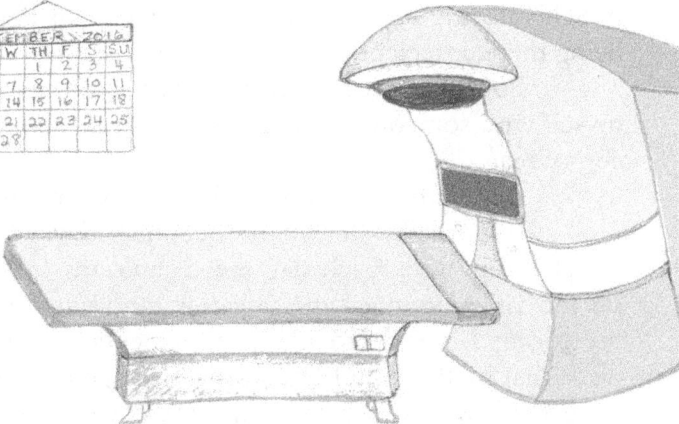

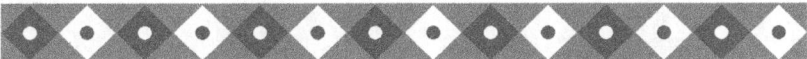

77

How to — Image Your Way Through Radiation

The first day of radiation was like being in the middle of Star Wars. They helped me off the table at the end of it and I said, "I'm not sure I can do this twenty-four more days." They reassured me that I could.

Once home I called a friend and related to him the Star Wars atmosphere and my anxieties. Together we brainstormed. How could I get through it? What could I do? Where could I find help?

We devised five things to do:

First, I would count my breaths—not deep breathing because that interfered with what the technicians were doing and counted as movement and I was not to move. Just gentle breathing—up to twenty.

Second, I would visit a memory. I was to remember being there and to imagine actually being back there again. I started a list of memories I could use.

Third, I would choose a Jesus story and insert myself into the story—think of the details of that story, being there, interacting with the various people.

Fourth, I would create a new memory—image myself with someone I'd like to sit down with and have a cup of tea.

And fifth, I would sing chants inside my head.

It worked. For twenty-four more days it worked unbelievably well. Each day the technicians located me on the table, arranged the radiation, and when they left the room, I went into my five elements. I got to the place that by the time I had finished the gentle breathing I was ready and willing to go into the imagination and let them transport me.

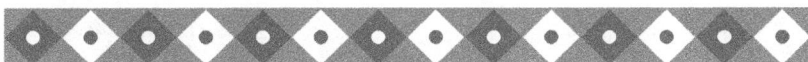

I went back to my 1995 visit to the Grand Canyon, I was in the Mary and Martha story, and I had a cup of tea and an amazing conversation with Thich Nhat Hanh, where he asked me a question and I answered him. I sang. I chanted. All silently and inside my head, but usually when the technicians came back in the room and said, "You're done Ms. Price," I could smile and say, "It was good."

Each day I used one chant over and over where I had written the music, and the words came from *The Message* by John H. Peterson, Joshua 1:9————Strength, courage, don't be timid. Don't be discouraged. God your God is with you every step you take.

I sing it still. It was true on those days of radiation and it still is.

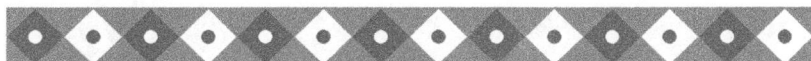

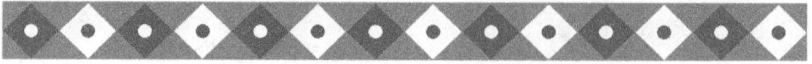

The Radiation Group

We're awaiting radiation every single day,
We're exchanging information and laughs along the way.
We are counting days 'till finished, 'till we ring that gong,
And we're doing it together—all the way along.

We became a group,
We became a group,
We became a radiation group.
Telling stories short,
Telling stories long,
We're a radiation group.

Maybe we will stay in touch,
Maybe we will let it go,
Either way it's been supportive -
The radiation group we know.

(Sing to the tune: I've Been Working on the Railroad)

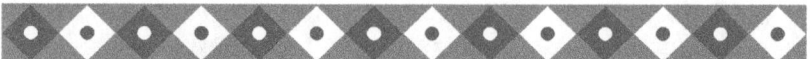

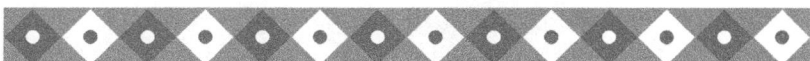

How to -- Eat

I'm not giving too many specifics because I am still figuring out my new food program, but I will say this: do some research on what you're eating. I have become convinced that some of the foods I used to eat contributed to the development of cancer in the first place and to the return of cancer a second and third time.

I now believe that what you eat is important for other diseases also.

This "how to" primarily is advising that if you have had cancer it is an excellent thing to check with someone who knows a lot about nutrition. You may have to try two or three nutritionists to find one that you can really do the work with. And keep doing your own research, and make the decisions to eat the best foods you can.

I have found some of Dr. Andrew Weil's books helpful.

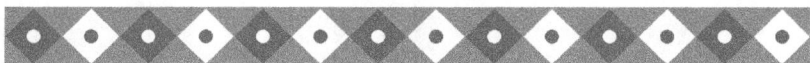

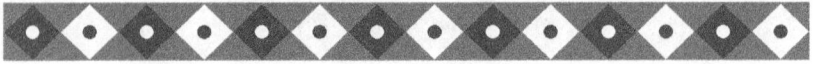

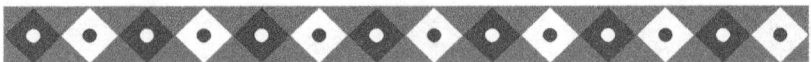

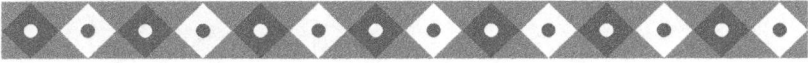

More Joy

Living

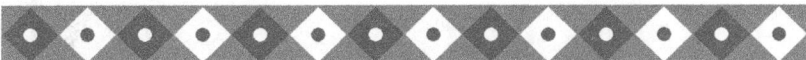

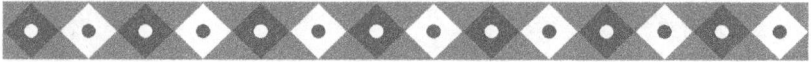

Sing

Sing as you walk
The road life's given you,
As you sing, remember
Angels sing with you.

You're not alone
For God is singing too,
What a chorus to be in,
Sing out, sing true.

(Sing to the tune: White Coral Bells)

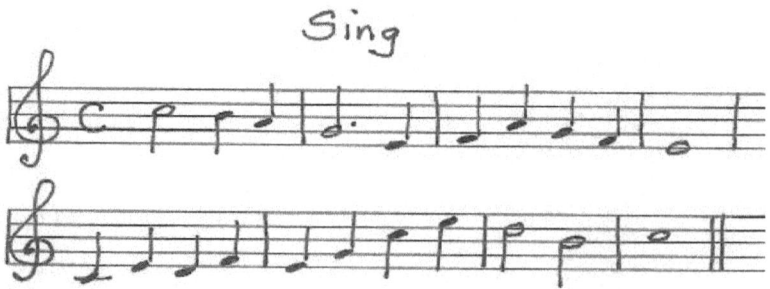

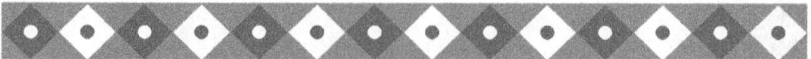

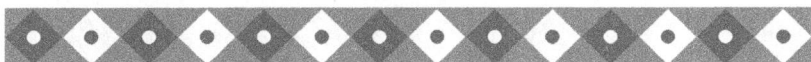

How to——Use Your Faith

My faith is woven throughout this book. Now at the conclusion of these fifteen years following the discovery of three cancers. Now after two lumpectomies and one left-side mastectomy. Now after chemo and twenty-five sessions of radiation, I know that I was never, ever alone. God was with me.

At the very beginning of the book of Joshua, Moses has died and in the first nine verses God speaks to Joshua. In Eugene Peterson's translation called The Message the words in the ninth verse are "Strength! Courage! Don't be timid. Don't be discouraged. God, your God, is with you every step you take!"

I believe that and I try to live it every day. I include here the chant that I wrote to those words and sang throughout this third episode of cancer.

Your faith can be your best encourager. Use it—in prayer, in song, in love and know that God walks with you. God certainly has walked this road with me.

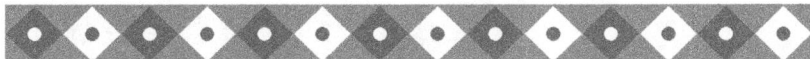

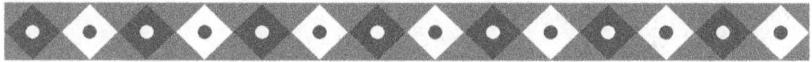

Strength! Courage!

Words: Joshua 1:9

Music: Ann Freeman Price

Music Copyright © 2016 Ann Freeman Price
Words: The Message

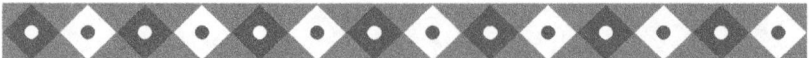

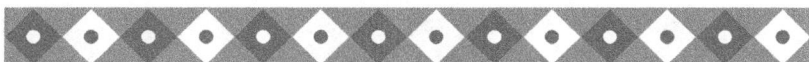

How to - Work Yoga Into Your Life

In May of 2018 my surgeon, Dr. Capko, officially said I could call if I needed to but I didn't need to come see her anymore. I continue to see my oncologist, Dr. Legresti, so I'm still making the trip to Sloan Kettering at least twice a year.
But in July of 2018 a new element entered my life which is making a healthy difference. I'm practicing yoga.

Here's what I think it's doing—it's helping my immune system, it's helping parts of my body that had become inflexible to be flexible again, it's helping me relax in meditation, it's helping me breathe in new and different ways.

I made a visit to the Himalayan Institute for a consultation with their doctor, Dr. Carrie Demers, and we created a continuing healing plan for me——and that plan includes yoga.

I've done individual sessions, I've done group sessions, I read books, I try things out and what I have discovered is that yoga is now a part of my life. What I do now at age 85 doesn't match the pictures in the books but you can see the concept there.

My meditation and my breathing do begin to match what the books describe.

Yoga is an ancient art and I make room for it—a little in the morning, a little more in the afternoon, and shavasana before bed. I have to admit that I look forward most of the day to that particular shavasana.

Thank you to all those who have gone before me in yoga and I look forward to continuing to make room for it each day for the rest of my life.

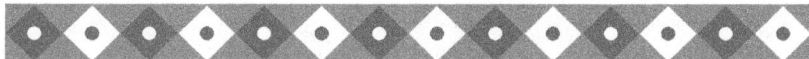

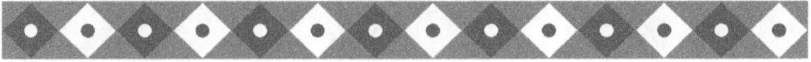

I Am Alive

Take a look around and I can see
Little bits of sky, a bird, a tree,
I am alive, yes I am alive and
Glad as I can be.

Never paid attention, now I do,
Family and friends I love, it's true,
I am alive, yes I am alive and
Every day is new.

Don't put off the words I want to say,
Make the minutes count in every way,
I am alive, yes I am alive and
Living every day.

(Sing to the tune: Kookaburra)

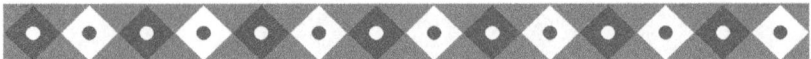

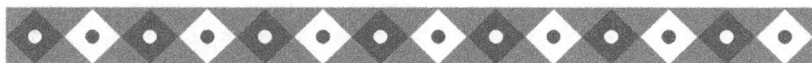

I Am Alive

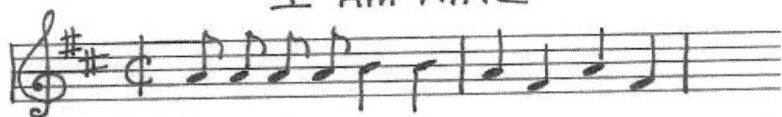

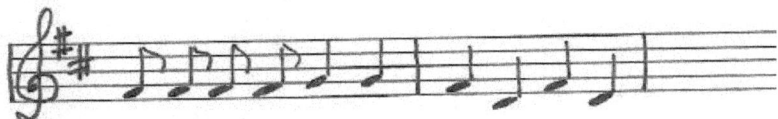

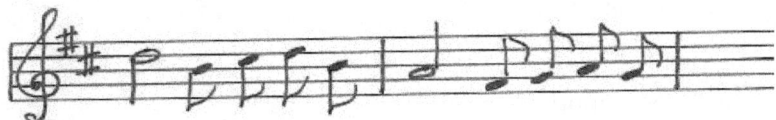

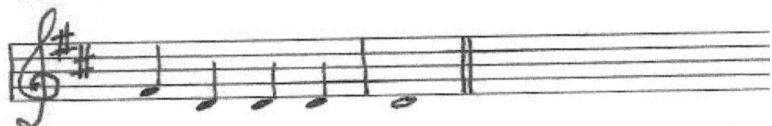

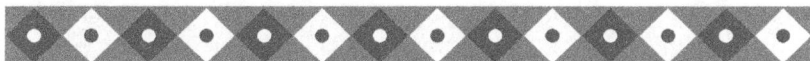

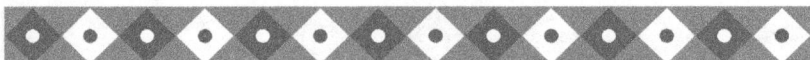

Each Day

live alive
alive to live
jokes to tell
gifts to give

time for serious
and silly time
rocks to hunt
hurdles to climb

silence and sound
conspire to shout
"life's a hoot !
live it out !"

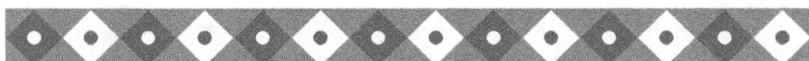

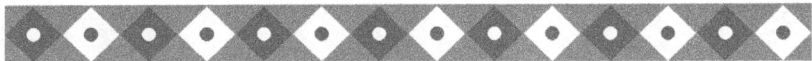

Thank You

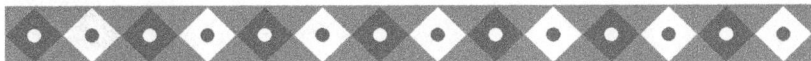

Thank You

Thank you's are part of the story.

I would say thank you to my family---four adult children and their partners, 16 grandchildren, and my former husband and his wife. These are the people who were initially dismayed at the diagnosis but then joined me on the journey. Each found significant ways to be supportive---varied and unique to them.

Friends near and far also found ways to be present---in person, by phone, by email, by sending things for my chemo notebook, by prayer.

At Sparta United Methodist Church my pastor, Charlie McNeil, gave counsel, friendship and met me at Memorial Sloan Kettering at 6am (a two hour trip), and twelve years later my pastor, Janice Sutton Lynn, made the same trip at a more reasonable time.

I had attended Sparta Church for only a month when I got the news of the first cancer. Even so, by then a host of friends plus those I barely knew surrounded me with care.

Those at Sloan Kettering---surgeons, music therapist, writing therapist, oncologists, radiologists, nurses, receptionists,---gave and continue to give their best skill and attention.

My radiation group, Angelique, Diane, Kim and Pura, helped me get from Day 1 to Day 25 of treatments.

I say thank you to all of these and to my God who promises to love---no exceptions.

This book is an optimistic book. Parts of the journey were hard but tucked in my life throughout is joy---and that's where I live now.

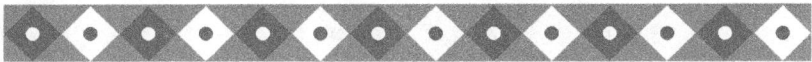

Ann
Freeman
Price

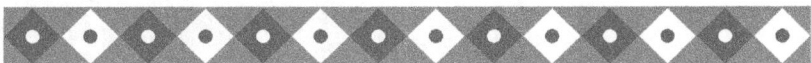

Ann Freeman Price

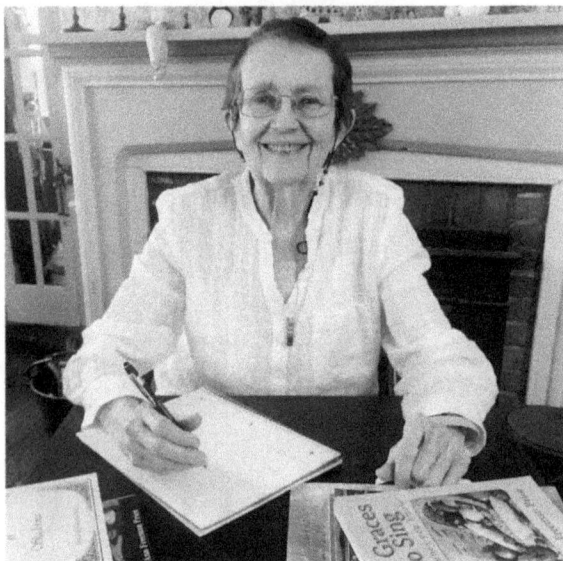

Ann Freeman Price is a writer and inspirational speaker.

She has had a variety of careers. She worked as a music therapist with the elderly for twelve years, and as a choir director and organist for fifteen. She served as a local pastor for a decade, first in the American Baptist Church and then in the United Methodist Church.

She has written church school curriculum for a variety of denominations and has published articles and poems in numerous magazines. She has led writing workshops called "Writing Down the Stories of Your Life," two of which lasted over a decade.

She created a cassette tape of songs she wrote and performed, titled "Woman Songs," which was then transformed into a stage musical at Belfry Repertory Company in

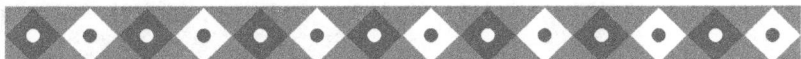

Nyack, NY. This cassette tape was then converted to a CD and is reissued on CDBaby.

She has written five other books: Mama and Me—Our Journey Together Her Last Three Years and Beyond; The Psalms in Shadorma; Wisdom of Children—Questions for God; 50 Graces to Sing to Tunes You Know, and a children's book: Do You Love Me? said the Grandchild to the Grandma, which was illustrated by her granddaughter Lissa Siew.

She is currently working on a Daybook of Personal Faith.

She received a Bachelors Degree from Butler University, Indianapolis, Indiana, the equivalent of a bachelors level major in music composition at Marymount College, Tarrytown, NY, and a Masters in Music Therapy degree from New York University.

She is a mother of four children (and their spouses), a grandmother of sixteen, has dabbled in clowning, juggles three balls, and on occasion has eaten fire.

Ann is 85 now and relishes opposites: time with people | time alone; reading | playing games alone or with others; thinking | doing; and trying to figure out on a daily basis what God wants her to do. She welcomes your comments.

You can reach her through her website:

AnnFreemanPrice.com

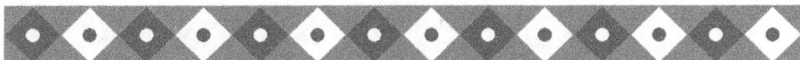

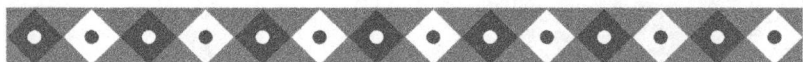

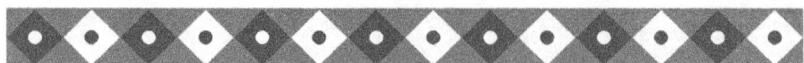

www.ingramcontent.com/pod-product-compliance
Lightning Source LLC
Chambersburg PA
CBHW031437270326
41930CB00007B/753